CARE ADVOCATES™
CARE OPTIONS • SENIOR PLACEMENT

CREATING A CARE (GIVING) PLAN

GUIDING YOUR CARE JOURNEY: HOW TO CREATE A PERSONALIZED CAREGIVING PLAN

Laura Daniels, BSN, RN, CCM

TABLE OF CONTENTS

INTRODUCTION 04

EIGHT TOPICS TO EXPLORE BEFORE CREATING A CARE PLAN 06

1. START THE CONVERSATION 06
2. ASSESS THE CURRENT SITUATION. 08
3. REVIEW YOUR LOVED ONE'S FINANCES. 08
4. END OF LIFE PLANNING AND PREFERENCES 10
5. AGING IN PLACE. 11
6. CONSIDER ASSISTED LIVING AND CARE OPTIONS OUTSIDE THE HOME. 11
7. CREATE YOUR CARE TEAM. 12
8. CARING FOR YOURSELF THE CAREGIVER. 13

EIGHT THINGS TO CONSIER WHEN CREATING A CARE (GIVING) PLAN FOR YOUR LOVED ONE. 15

1. ADDRESSING PHYSICAL & MENTAL HEALTH NEEDS IN A CARE P, ... 15
2. ADDRESSING YOUR LOVED ONE'S HEALTH NEEDS. 16
3. ASSESSING YOUR LOVED ONE'S ABILITY TO MANAGE FINANCES. 17
4. ADDRESSING YOUR LOVED ONE'S LEGAL MATTERS. 17
5. ENSURING YOUR LOVED ONE'S SAFETY AT HOME. 18
6. ASSESSING YOUR LOVED ONE'S SOCIAL & LIFESTYLE NEEDS. 19
7. INVOLVING YOUR LOVED ONE IN THEIR CARE PLAN. 20
8. CREATING YOUR CAREGIVING TEAM & SUPPORT SYSTEM FOR A CARE PLAN. 21

DEVELOPING YOUR CARE PLAN. 23

HELPFUL GLOSSARY YOU WILL NEED 25

RESOURCES 32

WORKSHEET 39

1. GOALS & NEEDS CHECKLIST. 39
2. GENERAL NEEDS ASSESSMENT. 40
3. PERSONAL INFORMATION CHECKLIST. 42
4. HOME MAINTENANCE CHECKLIST. 43
5. MEDICAL CHECKLIST. 44
6. MEDICAL CHECKLIST (CONTINUED). 46
7. LIST OF MEDICATIONS. 47
8. TRANSPORTATION CHECKLIST. 48
9. FINANCIAL ITEM CHECKLIST. 49
10. BENEFITS CHECKLIST. 50
11. CAREGIVING PLAN. 51
12. SAMPLE DETAILED FOR TASKS. 52

RESOURCES, ADVOCACY, GUIDANCE, SUPPORT 53

INTRODUCTION

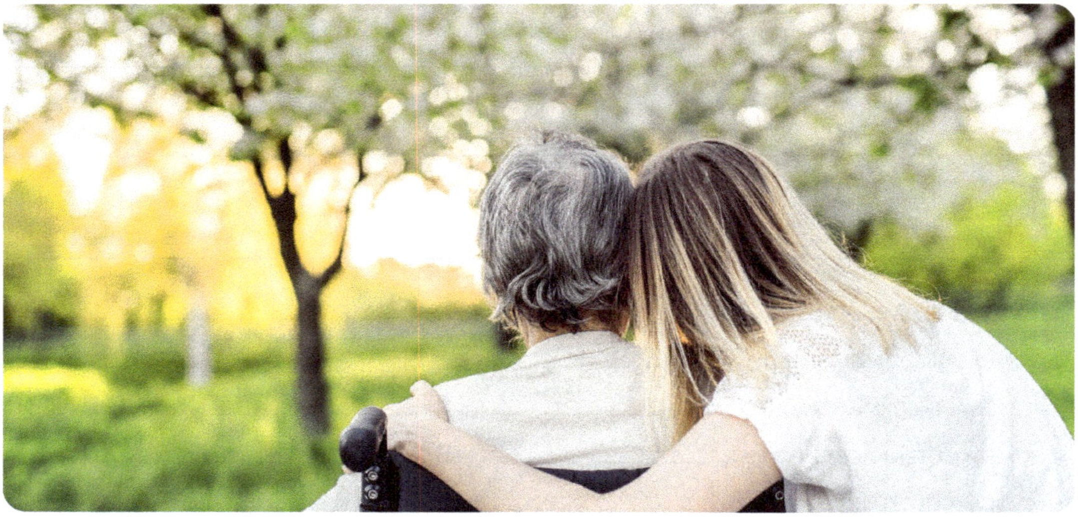

Caring for a loved one or a family member is one of the most important roles you will have. You may begin by driving your loved ones to the grocery store or to see the doctor. You may later find yourself spending more time at home, cooking meals, or paying bills.

You and your loved ones will find it easier to navigate the caregiving journey if you have a framework to guide you. This guide can help you provide care for yourself or a loved one. This guide will provide you with information, checklists, and resources to help you become organized and find support.

WHAT IS A CARE PLAN?

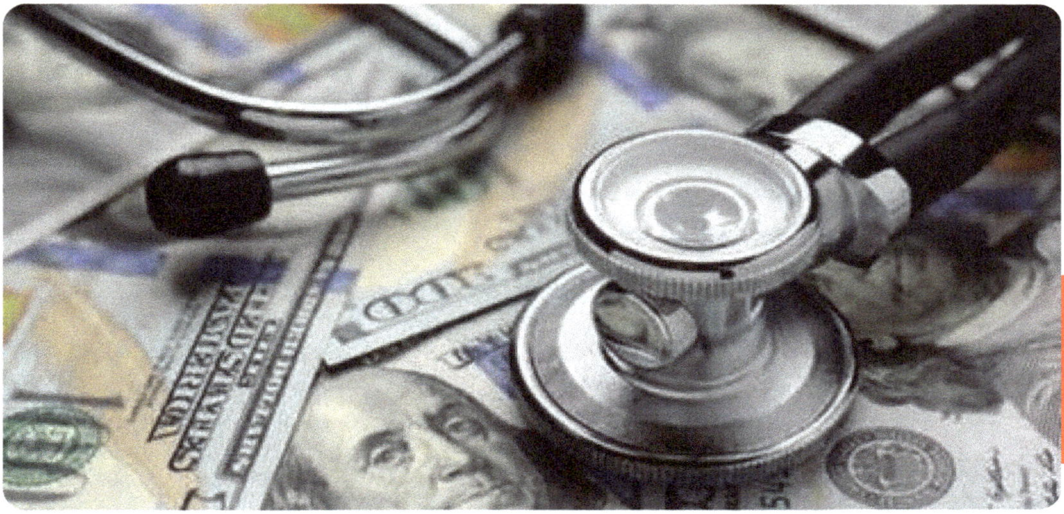

A care plan outlines your loved one's care needs.It promotes better health, safety, and quality of life. Care plans are different from a plan of care, which your loved one's doctor typically provides. A care (giving) plan helps you prepare for non-medical needs, arrange outside care support, and prepares you for future care transition and personal needs. This can lead to better communication, safe planning, and less stress.

At some point, most older adults will need help getting through the day. This means requiring assistance with basic living activities such as personal care, bathing, dressing, walking and toileting. Medicare typically does not pay for long-term care (typically called custodial care). Most families do not begin planning for this type of care until they are faced with a health crisis. This can lead to unnecessary stress, disagreements, and rising expenses that can happen from not preparing for future care needs.

Having a care plan well in advance allows families to get organized, locate appropriate resources and be prepared before a crisis hits. "A care plan is thinking through every step of what you or your loved one is going to need as you age, to ensure safety and preparedness," Laura Daniels says.

EIGHT TOPICS TO EXPLORE BEFORE CREATING A CARE PLAN

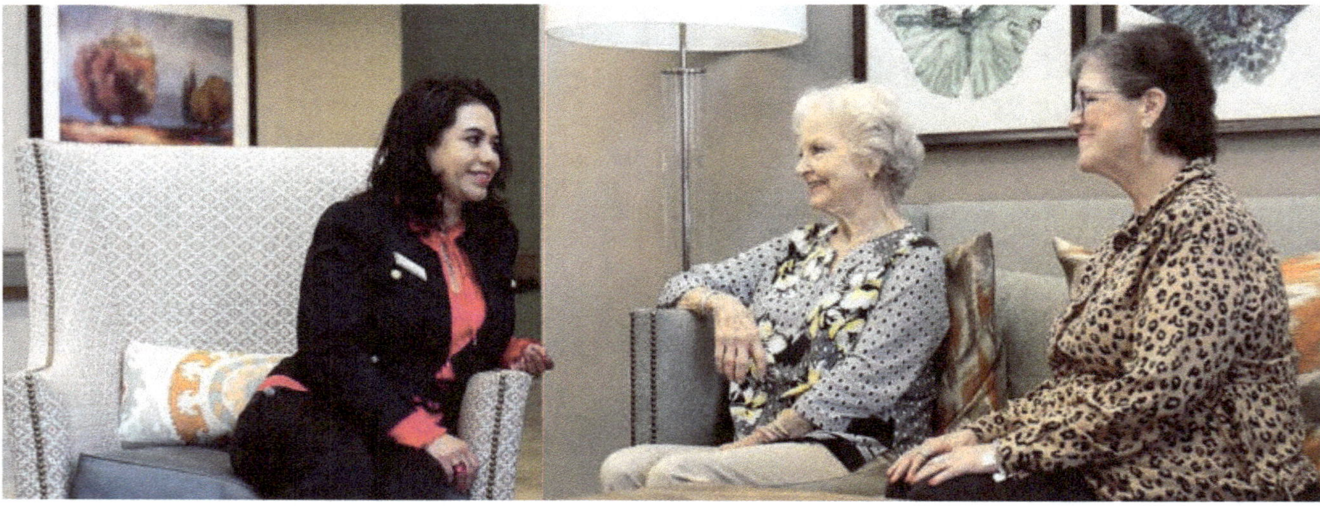

01. Start the Conversation About Care Planning Today

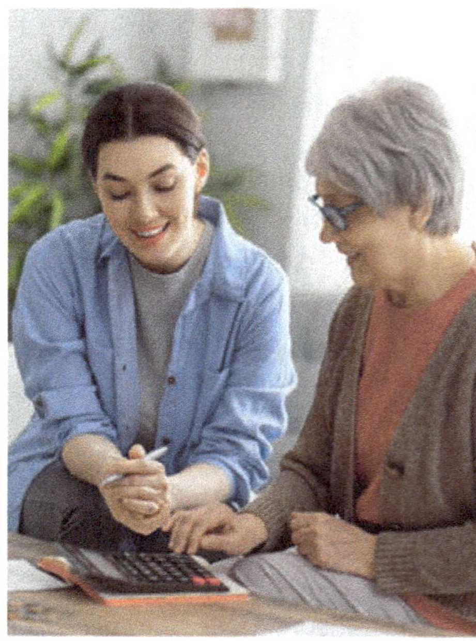

Start the conversation. People often wait for a crisis to occur before discussing their values, preferences, health care wishes or financial details. Waiting until you or your loved one have a serious accident, a fall or a diagnosis to make big decisions can lead to assumptions, anxiety and stress.

You can avoid a lot of anxiety by talking to your loved ones before anything happens. These conversations can be hard, so it's easy for us to delay them. We never feel like it's the right moment to discuss a topic we believe will be uncomfortable. It may surprise you to learn that your loved ones have been wanting to talk about the topic for a while.

Find an opportunity to begin this important conversation. Use an article or news item that you have read to bring up the subject of future care and creating a care (giving) plan that helps you prepare.

Some ideas for conversation starters with your loved ones:

1. You mentioned that your knees were bothering you. Does this cause problems when you are walking around the house or driving?

2. I just read an interesting article on how to gather all your important documents. You can show me yours and tell usadvise what to do in the event of an emergency.

3. If you want to consider staying in the house for a while. The the stairs could be a problem."

4. You were complaining about your vision. Do you have any problems with your eyesight when reading or driving?

Respect the wishes of your loved ones. Respect the wishes of your loved one. It is important to never make a care plan without your loved ones' participation, consent and knowledge. Persons with cognitive impairments should be included as much as they can.

You may want to invite a few trusted family members and friends to join the discussion once you have started it.You and your family members should discuss the following before meeting.

- Who's the best person for starting or leading the conversation?
- What is the best way to describe your feelings and thoughts about this situation?
- What are you hoping to accomplish or what do you think the best possible outcome will be as a result?
- What are the things you're prepared and unprepared to do?
- What is the most difficult part of having this conversation?

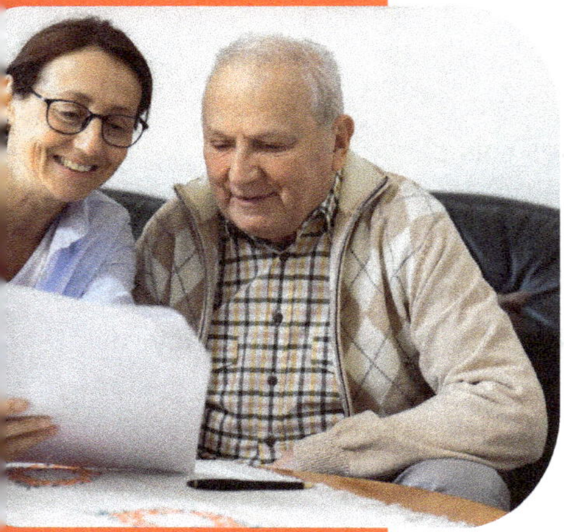

02. Assess the current situation

Start the conversation. People often wait for a crisis to occur before discussing their values, preferences, health care wishes or financial details. Waiting until you or your loved one have a serious accident, a fall or a diagnosis to make big decisions can lead to assumptions, anxiety and stress.

You can avoid a lot of anxiety by talking to your loved ones before anything happens. These conversations can be hard, so it's easy for us to delay them. We never feel like it's the right moment to discuss a topic we believe will be uncomfortable. It may surprise you to learn that your loved ones have been wanting to talk about the topic for a while.

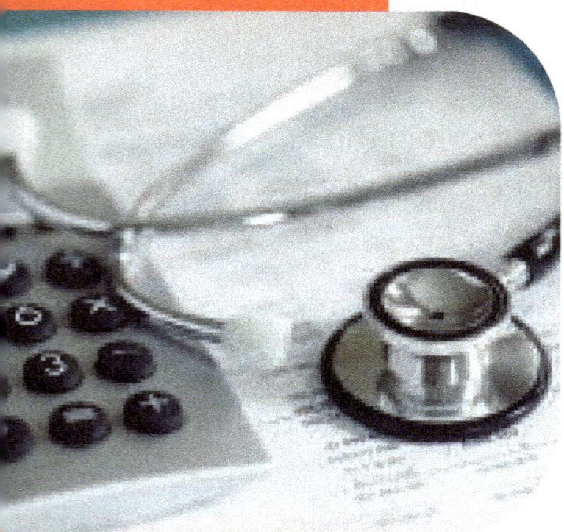

03. Review your loved one's finances

Examine finances. Money may be sensitive subject, but it will play a key role in many decisions you'll need to make with your loved one about housing, healthcare and other expenses. Family caregivers may find it surprising that most health insurance policies like Medicare cover very little or none of the costs of care provided at nursing homes or assisted living residences, or through daily activities such as bathing, dressing, or eating support services.

Find out if they have investments, insurance coverage and loans available that may cover potential care needs. Furthermore, inquire as to long-term care insurance and assets that could potentially cover potential care needs.

What is your loved one's income? Does your loved one have savings? Does your loved one have long-term care insurance or can they get a reverse mortgage? Will other family members assist with care expenses? Does your loved one qualify for government help, such as veteran's benefits, Medicaid or state programs? Do you know how to plan ahead for future care needs? These are all difficult questions, but they are vital and important.

Traditionally, Medicare does not cover the costs of assisted living or long-term care. There are several ways to pay for long-term care needs:

1. VA benefits for veterans and spouses of veterans who have served at least 90 days on active duty and at least one day during wartime. Applicants must meet a medical qualification test, but their conditions don't need to be related to military service.

2. Long-term care insurance. Less than 5% of families are fortunate enough to have long term-care insurance. These individuals use those financial benefits to help with the cost of assisted living.

3. Medicaid. Must qualify financially for medical.

4. Private pay. A majority of long-term care is privately paid by the individual needing care of their family.

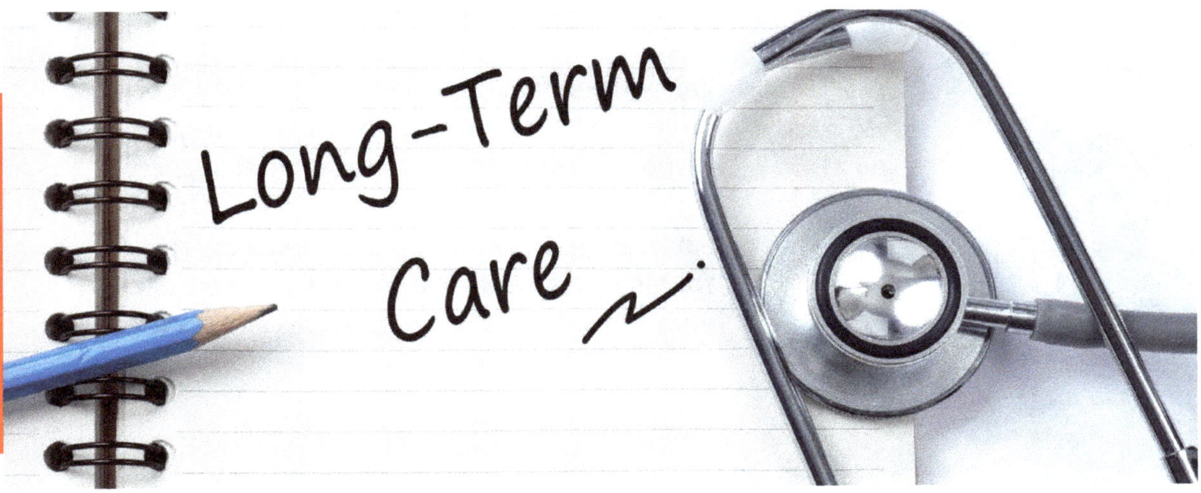

04. End of Life Planning and Preferences

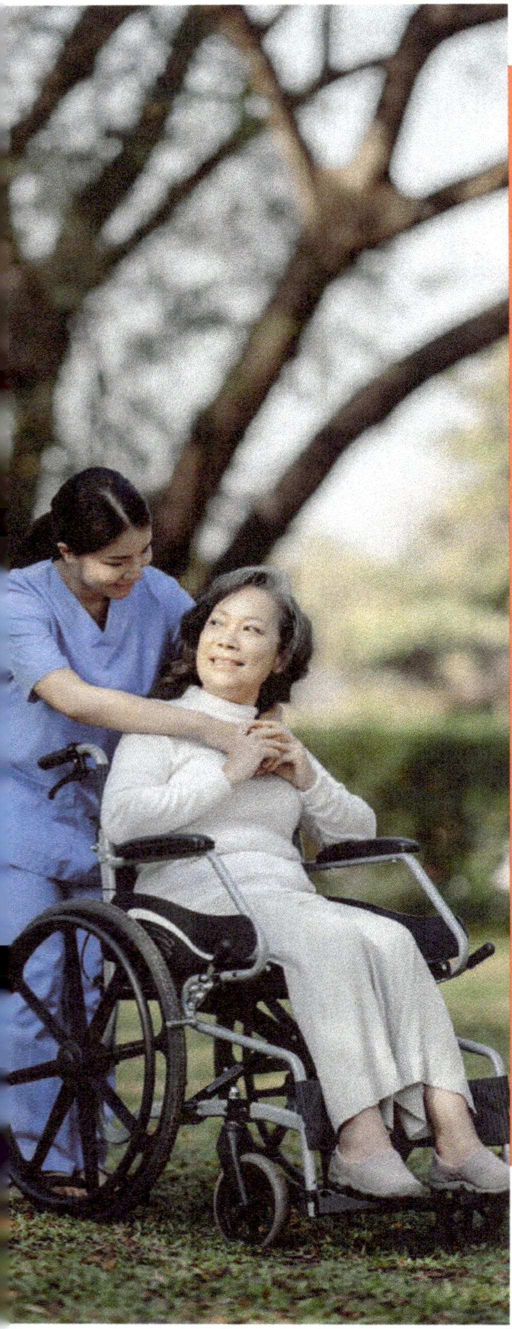

Having a open discusstion about end-of-life planning ensures that a loved one's wishes, comfort, and dignity are respected in their final stage of life. It involves establishing advance directives and legal documents, such as a Living Will, Healthcare Power of Attorney (POA), and DNR/DNI orders, to outline medical preferences.

Pain management and comfort care, including palliative or hospice care, help focus on symptom relief and quality of life. Emotional and psychological support, such as counseling, life review activities, and meaningful goodbyes, can provide reassurance and closure.

Spiritual and religious considerations should be honored, allowing for faith-based rituals, beliefs, and support from spiritual leaders. Financial and estate planning, including wills, trusts, and funeral preferences, helps ensure that assets are handled according to their wishes.

Lastly, open family communication and support are essential, with discussions about roles, responsibilities, and planning for grief support.

Addressing these aspects early reduces stress for family members and ensures that care aligns with a loved one's personal values and choices.

05. Aging in place

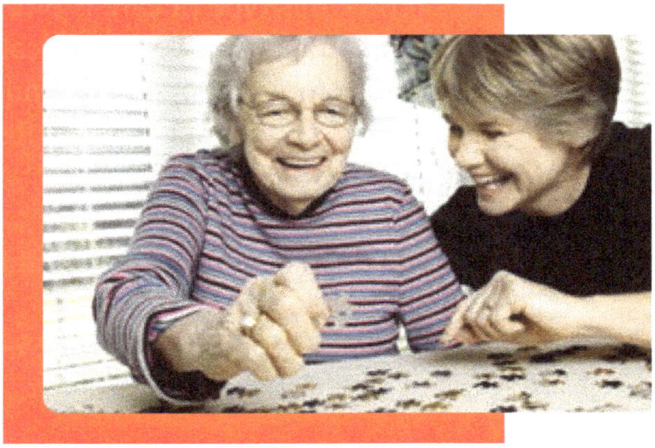

Almost everyone wants prefers to stay in their home as they age, something called "aging in place." This means relying on family members for care, or paid in- homein-home care (caregivers in your the home). This can get expensive quickly. Nationally, a full-time caregiver 24 hours per day in 2024 is $20,740 per month. That is the national average. There can be a lot of variation between states, According according to the Genworth Cost of Care Survey, .

Adaptations can allow an older person to remain in the home if they're disabled. Some changes might be simple, such as removing throw rugs that could cause falls, remove clutter and reorganizing their living space. Other changes like widening doorways or modifying a shower can get expensive. The sooner you get this evaluation, the more time you will have to plan and pay for this.

06. Consider assisted living and care options outside the home

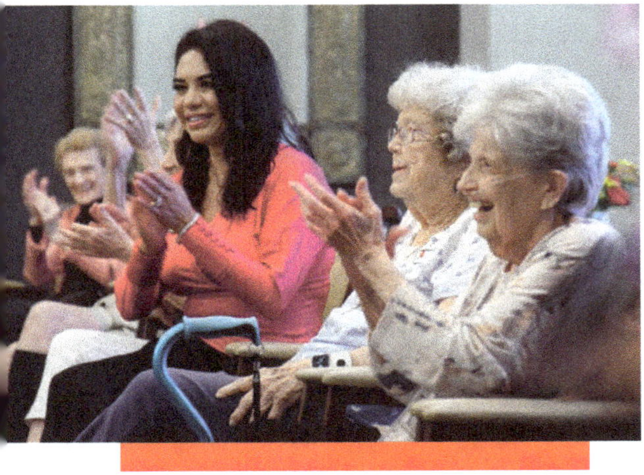

Even if the home supports aging in place, other factors might not support this. Consider how the older person will socialize, be socially engaged, get groceries and make it to health appointments if they can no longer drive. An independent living or senior living community could provide more amenities, companionship, care and safety.

If you have been concerned about your aging parent or loved one living on their own, you may want to explore senior living options for their care and safety. Researching this type of care is often a new concept for many families. When we are talking about senior care, typically we are talking about five distinct types of care options for your loved one: Independent Living, Assisted Living, Memory Care, Respite Care and Skilled Nursing. Researching these and having a plan in place is another step to complete.

For more detailed information contact me, your local Care Advocate:

Laura Daniels, BSN, RN at 210-669-2222 or https://advocatern.com/.

07. Create your Care Team

A caregiving team is needed to support you and your loved one. The extra support ensures your loved one's care needs are consistently met, even when you're unavailable. It also gives you an opportunity for respite care when necessary. Your care team should designate one person for each area of your loved one's care. They won't be responsible for every task that falls in their category, but they will ensure that each one is completed.

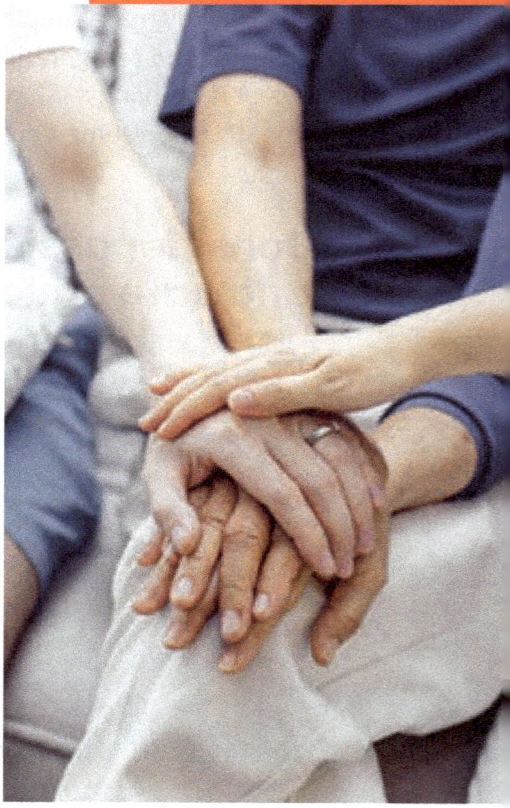

Nobody should take on the responsibility of caring for someone alone. Other family members may be sources of help, but don't ignore friends, co-workers, clubs, religious or other affiliations. It's okay to ask for help. You can get help from a local organizations and resources if the care required is greater than what you and your team are able to provide.
https://advocatern.com/resources/

Community resources are available. Many age-related support services are available for people of all ages. You can find out about services like adult day service centers, home delivered meals, transportation and care management. Visit www.eldercare.gov to find out what services are available in your area.

Consult a local elder care professional at to streamline the search and locate the right resources and care needed, at https://advocatern.com/. Many times, the needs of a loved-oneloved one can be complicated, especially when emotional, financial, and health issues are involved. An elder care professional can help you identify what's needed, locate services, arrange care, and access all care options and Medicare covered resources.

08. Caring for yourself, the caregiver

This is probably one of the most important topics. You must take care of yourself before you can advocate for and care for those you love. Do not underestimate the impact that caregiving has on you. It can be difficult to balance caregiving and work with other obligations. Families who care for others often mention that the hardest part is balancing work and family obligations because of the demand for their time.

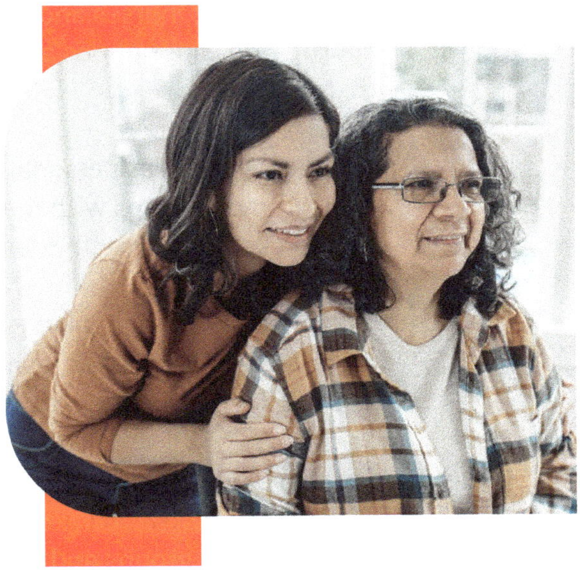

The demand for their time. Stress can have a negative impact on your health, wellbeing and ability to care for others. Plan regular time to do what you enjoy and ask for help.

Recognize the emotions you feel. You may feel differently about your experience depending on how you got involved as a caretaker. If you've always felt close to your loved ones, you may see the role as a way to return their loving care. Others might have felt resentful at being forced to shoulder the responsibility because of their work, family and own responsibilities. Some people enter caregiving reluctantly. They may find that it is a great opportunity to heal a distant or broken relationship. It doesn't matter how you got into this role, but it is important to understand your emotions.

Take good care of yourself. Pay attention to your personal needs, such as exercise, healthy eating and sleep. Take time to enjoy yourself and find ways to reduce stress. When you care for yourself, you are often better equipped to take care of your loved one. To cope, consider tapping into social networks.

Coordinating care when you live outside the community can be expensive, frustrating and time-consuming. You can use the following resources and techniques to help you:

- Social workers, nurses and other professionals can guide you in selecting appropriate care options and monitoring their delivery when you live far away from them.

- Technology such as personal emergency response systems, remote monitoring devices, mobile apps with medical records and electronic calendar reminders can assist in keeping up with the many tasks necessary for long-distance caregivers.

- Organization is essential when caring long distance - keeping a list of contact info for doctors, insurance companies and neighbors, including medications they take - is also crucial to success in caregiving long distance.

- Creating and completing a caregiving care plan is the first start. Download a care giving plan worksheet/ needs assessment: https://advocatern.com/resources/ Many support groups and caring organizations exist. It can be comforting to know that you're not alone. You may find new ways to reduce the workload. You can get help from the community to care for others. Do not feel ashamed if you or your family member needs time to rest, or if you require help understanding information.

EIGHT THINGS TO CONSIER WHEN CREATING A CARE (GIVING) PLAN FOR YOUR LOVED ONE.

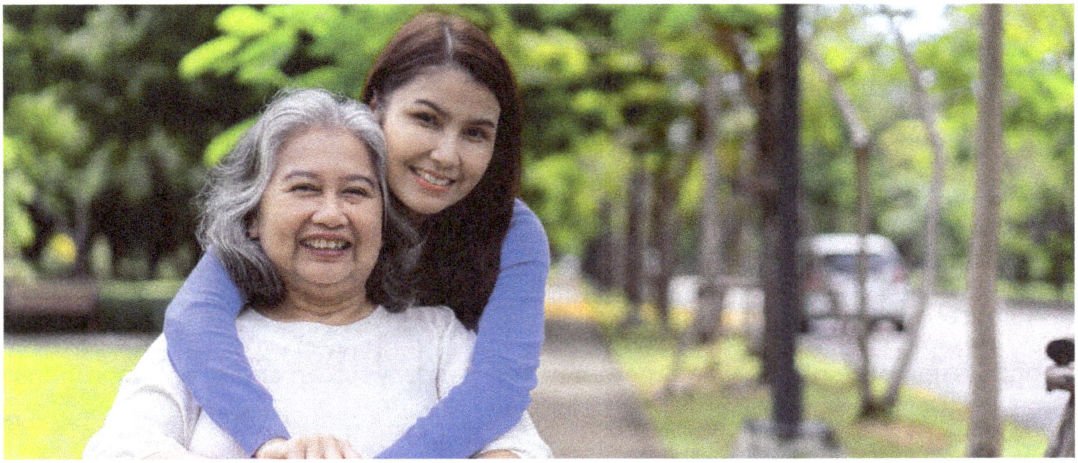

A well-rounded care plan should prioritize both physical and mental well-being by addressing key areas:

01. Addressing Physical & Mental Health Needs in a Care Plan

- **Mobility & Independence** – Assess mobility, prevent falls, and encourage light exercise.
- **Nutrition & Hydration** – Ensure a balanced diet, accommodate dietary needs, and promote hydration.
- **Personal Hygiene & Grooming** – Adapt routines with accessible modifications and assist as needed.
- **Medical & Medication Management** – Keep up with doctor visits, monitor chronic conditions, and ensure proper medication use.

- **Pain & Comfort** – Address pain concerns, provide comfortable furniture, and explore alternative therapies.
- **Sleep & Rest** – Maintain a consistent sleep schedule, create a restful environment, and manage sleep disturbances.
- **Daily Activities (ADLs)** – Assist with dressing, toileting, and eating while maintaining dignity.
- **Assessing Mental Health & Emotional Well-Being**
  - Monitor for signs of depression, anxiety, or cognitive decline.
  - Encourage social engagement through activities, visits, and hobbies.
  - Provide mental stimulation with games, puzzles, music, and storytelling.
  - Support emotional health by addressing fears, grief, or loneliness with open conversations and professional counseling if needed.

By addressing both physical and mental health needs, you can create a comprehensive care plan that promotes overall well-being, independence, and quality of life.

02. Addressing Your Loved One's Health Needs

- **Regular Medical Check-Ups** – Ensure they visit primary care doctors, specialists, and dentists regularly.
- **Medication Management** – Set up reminders, track prescriptions, and prevent medication errors.
- **Chronic Condition Care** – Develop a plan for managing conditions like diabetes, heart disease, or dementia.
- **Nutritional and Physical Health** – Ensure they have a balanced diet, regular exercise, and proper hydration.
- **Mental Health & Well-Being** – Monitor for signs of depression, anxiety, or cognitive decline and provide social engagement.
- **End-of-Life Preferences** – Discuss palliative care, hospice options, and medical decisions in advance.

03. Assessing Your Loved One's Ability to Manage Finances

- **Look for Signs of Financial Difficulty** – Missed bills, unusual spending, or susceptibility to scams.
- **Evaluate Financial Literacy** – Can they track expenses, manage income, and understand obligations?
- **Identify Cognitive or Physical Barriers** – Memory loss, difficulty handling transactions, or paperwork confusion.
- **Discuss Future Planning** – Ensure they have a financial power of attorney, long-term care plans, and estate documents.
- **Offer Support While Maintaining Independence** – Set up automated payments, involve a trusted advisor, and protect against financial exploitation.

By assessing these factors, you can help ensure their **financial stability and security** while preserving their **independence and dignity.**

04. Addressing Your Loved One's Legal Matters

- **Healthcare Power of Attorney (POA)** – Assign a trusted person to make medical decisions if they become unable.
- **Living Will or Advance Directive** – Document their medical treatment preferences and end-of-life care wishes.
- **Financial Power of Attorney (POA)** – Designate someone to manage finances, pay bills, and handle transactions.
- **Wills and Estate Planning** – Ensure assets, property, and personal belongings are legally designated.

- **Long-Term Care Planning** – Review insurance policies, Medicaid/Medicare options, and future care costs.
- **Protection Against Fraud & Scams** – Educate them on financial scams targeting seniors and safeguard their assets.
- **Legal Document Organization** – Keep copies of important legal paperwork accessible and up to date.

By proactively **managing health and legal concerns**, you help secure your loved one's **well-being, financial stability, and peace** of mind for the future.

05. Ensuring Your Loved One's Safety at Home

- **Fall Prevention** – Remove trip hazards, install grab bars, improve lighting, and use non-slip mats.
- **Mobility & Accessibility** – Arrange furniture for clear pathways, use assistive devices, and add ramps if needed.
- **Emergency Preparedness** – Install smoke detectors, post emergency numbers, and provide a medical alert system.
- **Kitchen Safety** – Use auto-shutoff appliances, store sharp objects safely, and monitor stove use.
- **Bathroom Safety** – Install grab bars, use a shower chair, and adjust water temperature to prevent burns.
- **Security & Fraud Protection** – Use door locks, security cameras, and educate on scam prevention.
- **Medication & Health Monitoring** – Organize medications, set reminders, and schedule regular health check-ins.

By making these **home safety improvements**, you can help your loved one live **securely and independently** while reducing risks.

06. Assessing Your Loved One's Social & Lifestyle Needs

- **Social Engagement** – Evaluate their connections, participation in community activities, and support network.
- **Hobbies & Interests** – Identify favorite pastimes and explore adaptive options to keep them engaged.
- **Daily Routine & Structure** – Ensure they have a balanced schedule with social, physical, and mental activities.
- **Emotional & Mental Well-Being** – Watch for signs of depression or anxiety and provide emotional support.
- **Technology & Communication** – Assess their ability to use phones, social media, or video calls to stay connected.
- **Transportation & Accessibility** – Determine if they can drive safely or need alternative transportation.
- **Purpose & Meaning** – Encourage volunteering, caregiving roles, or faith-based activities to give them a sense of purpose.
- **Cognitive Stimulation** – Incorporate puzzles, reading, or new learning experiences to maintain brain health.
- **Dining & Social Meals** – Address mealtime isolation and explore group dining options for companionship.
- **Religious & Spiritual Needs** – Support participation in faith-based services, prayer groups, or meditation.
- **Stress Management & Relaxation** – Introduce relaxation techniques like music, yoga, or mindfulness for emotional balance.

By addressing these key lifestyle factors, you can help your loved one stay socially connected, mentally engaged, and emotionally fulfilled, leading to a better quality of life.

07. Involving Your Loved One in Their Care Plan

- **Open Communication** – Have honest conversations about care preferences before a crisis occurs and listen to their concerns.
- **Encourage Decision-Making** – Use gentle questioning to assess comfort levels and start with small decisions(e.g., meal choices, routines) to build confidence in larger care-related choices.
- **Personalized Care Plan** – Tailor care to their physical, emotional, and social needs, incorporating their hobbies, interests, and values.
- **Respect Their Independence** – Support self-care and mobility while providing assistance only when needed.
- **Keep Them Informed** – Explain medical conditions, involve them in appointments, and document their preferences.
- **Identify Meaningful Relationships** – Ensure they stay connected with friends, family, and social circles that matter to them.
- **Build a Support System** – Engage family, caregivers, and peer communities for collaboration and emotional support.

By actively **involving your loved** one in their care plan, you empower them to **maintain independence, dignity**, and control over their well-being.

08. Creating Your Caregiving Team & Support System for a Care Plan

Building a **strong caregiving** team ensures your loved one receives well-rounded, consistent, and high-quality care. Here's how to create a **reliable support system:**

1. Identify Key Care Team Members

- **Family Members** – Define roles for family members (primary caregiver, financial manager, appointment coordinator).
- **Professional Caregivers** – Consider in-home caregivers, skilled nurses, or senior living staff.
- **Healthcare Providers** – Include doctors, specialists, therapists, and home health/hospice services.
- **Legal & Financial Advisors** – Consult attorneys for POA and estate planning, and financial planners for long-term care costs.
- **Community Support** – Leverage senior centers, faith-based groups, or volunteer services.

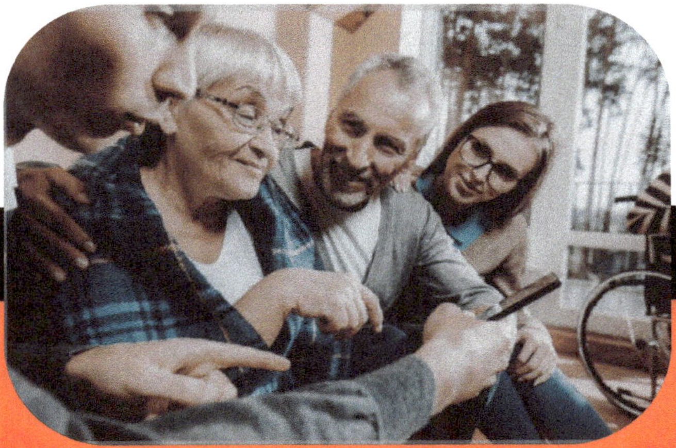

2. Assign Roles & Responsibilities

- Establish **clear tasks** for each caregiver (medical care, household chores, transportation, social visits).
- Use a **shared calendar or caregiving app** to coordinate schedules.
- Plan for **backup caregivers** in case of emergencies.

3. Foster Communication & Collaboration

- Hold **regular check-ins** with the care team to discuss updates and concerns.
- Ensure everyone understands your loved one's **care preferences and goals.**
- Keep a **care notebook** or digital log for medications, appointments, and important notes.

4. Utilize Community & Professional Resources

- Connect with **support groups** for caregivers.
- Explore **respite care options** to prevent burnout.
- Look into **Medicare, Medicaid, and veteran benefits** for additional assistance.

5. Adjust the Care Plan as Needs Change

- Reassess the care plan regularly to accommodate evolving health conditions.
- Stay flexible and be open to adding new team members or services.

By **building a strong caregiving team,** you create a **support system that ensures your loved one's needs are metwhile** preventing caregiver burnout and ensuring continuity of care.

DEVELOPING YOUR CARE PLAN

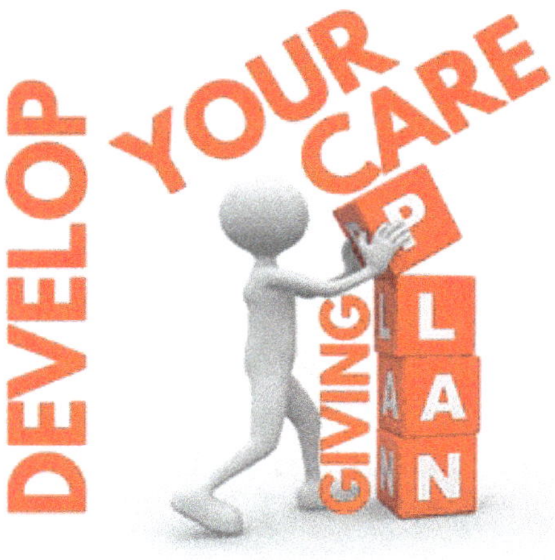

Once you have a care team and a reliable support system, you can move on to creating a plan. Not only should it account for your loved one's needs, but it should also address anyone else involved in their care.

A caregiver care plan should have:

- Contact information for your loved one's medical providers.
- The caregiving team's contact details and numbers.
- A schedule for your loved one's care.
- Your loved one's medication schedule and instructions.
- Critical medical information, such as health conditions, providers, allergies.
- Assigned responsibilities, such as "Laundry: Sally on Thursday afternoons."
- Instructions for any emergency that may occur.

CARRY OUT THE CARE PLAN

Once you have a plan, it's time to implement it. Make sure everyone involved in your loved one's care has a copy of the care plan. In addition, you should routinely consult your loved one's caregiving team and check on your loved one. As you receive new information about your loved one, including any changes, you can modify your plan so it continues to fit their needs. This paragraph is almost the same as the one at the end of this section.

Remember, a care plan is designed to simplify your responsibilities as a family caregiver. As you make revisions, don't forget to account for changes in your life. If you can't manage the workload as well as you initially thought, or it starts interfering with your physical, mental, and emotional health, then assign the task to somebody someone else.

Once you have a plan, write down the details and consider sharing it with family members or other people who may be involved in the care plan. It is important to revisit your plan, as circumstances can change over time. Planning your care as you age is not a one and done thing. It's an ongoing process. For more information and in-depth discussion of the areas addressed please visit advocateRN.com

For a free copy of a Care Plan Worksheet, visit

DOWNLOAD

HELPFUL GLOSSARY YOU WILL NEED

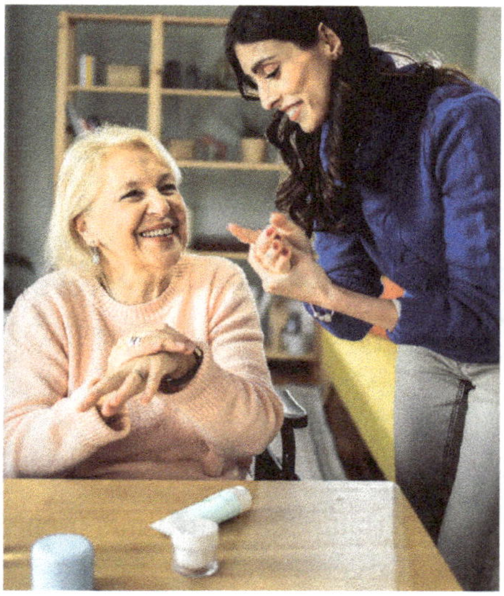

Activities of Daily Living (ADLs)

Basic tasks of everyday life that include, but are not limited to, dressing, bathing, eating and toileting.

Adult Day Services

Structured, comprehensive programs, including a variety of health, social and related support services during any part of the day but for less than 24 hours, provided at centers for adults who need some supervision and/or support.

Adult Protective Services

A public agency that investigates reports of abuse and neglect of vulnerable adults, usually working with law enforcement. Immediate dangerous situations should be directed to 911 or the local police.

Area Agency on Aging (AAA) or Aging and Disability Resource Center (ADRC)

An agency designated by the state with the responsibility for planning and coordinating services for older people or for older people and adults with disabilities within a specific geographical area. Both agencies provide information, resources, assistance and links to community services.

Assisted Living Residences

Housing for those who may need help living independently, but do not need skilled nursing care. The level of assistance varies among residences and may include help with bathing, dressing, meals and housekeeping.

Community Meal Program

Balanced, nutritious meals served at community locations for those age 60 and over and their spouses.

Conservator

A person appointed by a court to handle someone's affairs when that person cannot handle them him or herself. A conservator usually handles only financial affairs.

Continuing Care Retirement Communities

Housing that offers a variety of living options and services including independent living, assisted living and skilled care, often all on the same campus, designed to meet a person's changing needs.

Discharge Planner

A professional who assists individuals and their families in developing a plan of care for an individual following a hospital or nursing home stay.

DNR: Do Not Resuscitate Order

An order written by a doctor to fulfill an individual's expressed medical care wishes during a medical emergency.

Durable Power of Attorneyfor Finances

The durable power of attorney for finances is a legal document that allows you to give authority to another trusted person to make financial decisions on your behalf. The designation "durable" means that it will stay in effect if you become unable to manage your own financial affairs.

Elder Care Manager

Also known as a Geriatric Care Manager coordinates care between multiple service providers. Helps manage transitional care along with ongoing assessment of aging life care needs. For more information call 210-669-2222

Employee Assistance Program (EAP)

An employee benefit program offered by many employers. EAPs are intended to help employees deal with personal issues that affect their job performance, health and well-being. EAPs generally include short-term counseling and referral services for employees and their household members.

Family and Medical Leave Act

A law that requires some employers to let you take unpaid time off work (up to 12 weeks) for illness, having/adopting a baby, or caring for an ill family member. Your job or equivalent is guaranteed when you return. If you work for a small employer or are a new employee, you may not be able to get the leave

Family Caregiver

Anyone who provides unpaid assistance to another person who is ill, has a disability or needs help with daily activities.

Guardian

A person appointed by the court who is responsible for the care and management of another person who has been determined to be no longer capable of making decisions for him/herself.

Health Care Power of Attorney (HCPA Health Care Proxy)

A special kind of durable power of attorney in which you appoint another person to make health care decisions should you become unable to do so.

Health InsurancePortability and Accountability Act (HIPAA)

A federal law that gives you rights over your health information and sets rules and limits on who can look at and ook at and receive it. The law also permits the release of personal health information needed for patient care.

Home Health Agency

An agency often certified by Medicare to provide health-related services in the home such as nursing; occupational, speech, or physical therapy; social work and/or personal care.

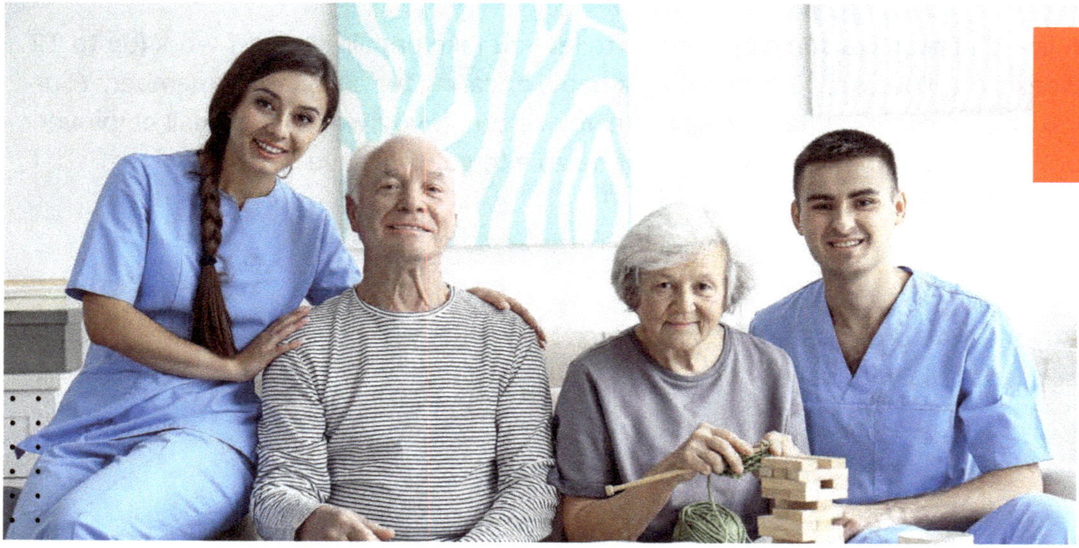

Home Health Aide

An individual who helps with bathing, dressing, grooming, assistance with meals, and light housekeeping.

Homemaker Services

A service that provides assistance with general household activities such as meal preparation, cleaning, laundry and shopping.

Instrumental Activities of Daily Living (IADL)

Professionally coordinated support services, including pain and symptom management, social services, and emotional and spiritual support for terminally ill people and their families. The care is provided at home and in other settings.

Continuing Care Retirement Communities

Basic tasks of everyday life that include, but are not limited to: managing money, shopping, telephone use, travel in the community, housekeeping, preparing meals and taking medications correctly.

Living Will (Part of a Health Care Directive)

A legal document that communicates a person's wishes about lifesaving medical treatments should he or she have a terminal condition and not be able to communicate their health care wishes.

Long-Term Care Insurance

Insurance that can pay part of the cost of care received in the home, assisted living residences, nursing home, and other designated services depending on the policy purchased.

Long-Term Care Ombudsman

A person who investigates and resolves complaints on behalf of residents of nursing homes and other long-term care facilities.

Medicare

A federal health insurance program for people age 65 and over, and for some younger people with disabilities. Medicare covers hospital stays, doctor visits, prescription drugs and other health care related needs. Medicare does not cover long-term care.

Medicare SavingsProgram

An assistance program for people with Medicare who need help with paying their Medicare expenses, such as premiums and possibly copays and deductibles for Medicare Parts A & B.

Medicaid

The federal/state-funded health and long-term care program for people with limited income and assets. It is administered by the states within federal guidelines, so eligibility and coverage may differ from state to state. For long-term care services, states have additional eligibility rules.

Nursing Home

A nursing facility that provides intermediate care, such as assistance with personal care and activities of daily living and/or skilled care; 24-hour medical, nursing and rehabilitation care; often a transition from hospital to home. The latter may be called a skilled nursing facility.

Palliative Care

Professionally coordinated services that focus on physical, mental, social and spiritual needs of those with life-threatening illness and their families. It seeks to maintain the highest level of comfort.

Personal EmergencyResponse System (PERS)

A portable electronic device with a call button that a person can use to summon help in an emergency.

Respite Care

A temporary break from providing care for a loved one. Respite care can be provided by family and/or friends through services such as attending an adult day services center. You can also have a paid home-care worker come to the home.

Social Security

A benefit earned by eligible workers that provides guaranteed inflation-adjusted monthly income for life. A person with the required number of quarters in Social Security is eligible at age 62 or if disabled. Certain family members may be eligible for benefits as well.

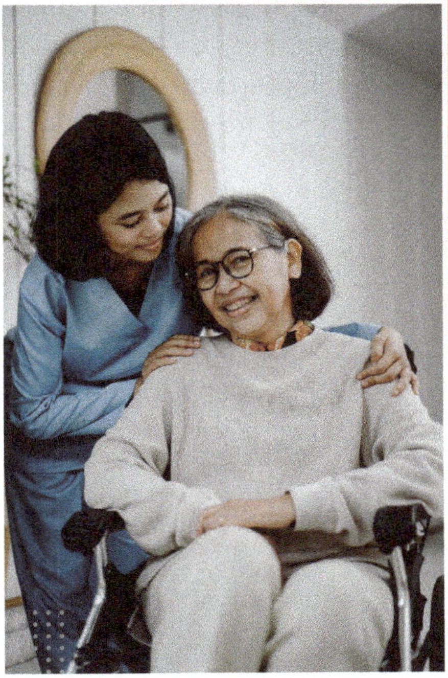

SupplementalSecurity Income (SSI)

SSI provides a monthly benefit to people who are 65 years of age and older, disabled or blind, and who have limited income and assets.

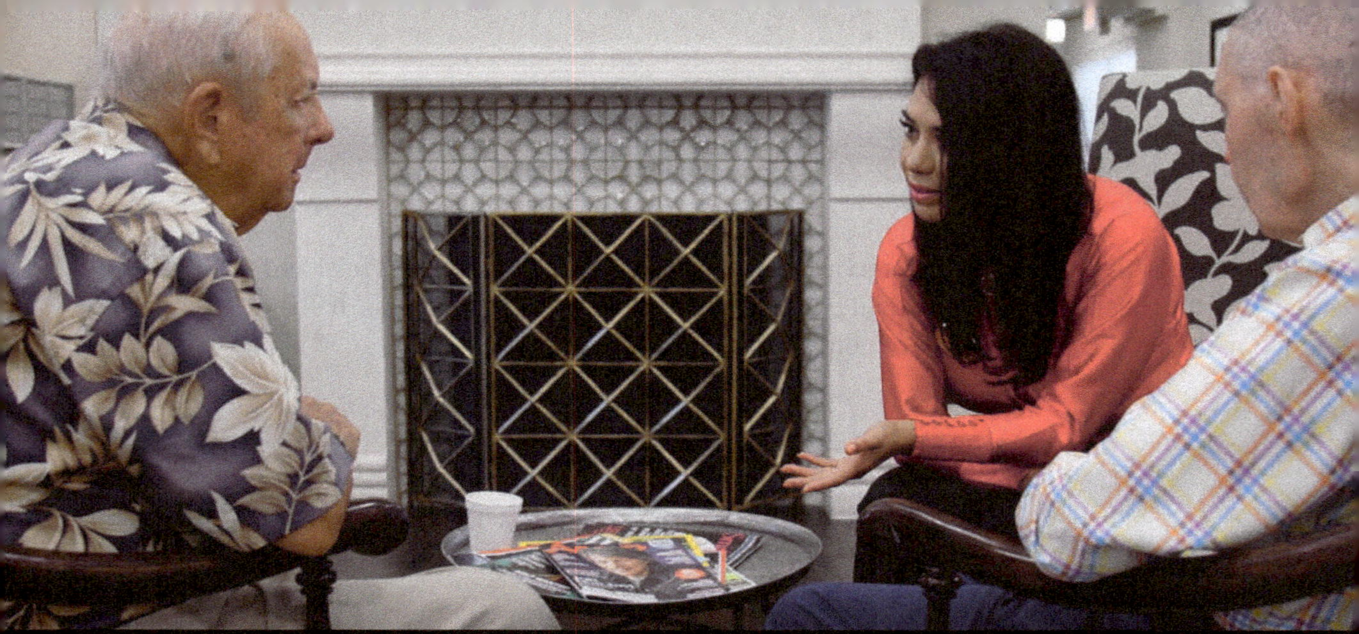

RESOURCES

AARP

AARP is a nonprofit membership organization dedicated to addressing the needs and interests of persons 50 and older. Site provides useful information and resources on topics such as: health and wellness; economic security and work; long-term care and independent living; and personal enrichment.

Website: http://www.aarp.org

AARP Caregiving Resource Center:

www.aarp.org/caregiving or 877-333-5885

A one-stop shop for tips, tools and resourceswhile caring for a loved one. For Spanish resourcesvisit www.aarp.org/cuidar or call 888-971-2013.

Advance DirectiveForms by State: www.aarp.org/careguides

Free, downloadable state-specific advance directiveforms and instructions.

AARP Care Guides: www.aarp.org/careguides

Take the stress out of caregiving with these targeted, easy-to-use guides.

AARP Local Caregiver Resource Guides:

www.aarp.org/caregiverresourceguides

Local resources that help make caregiving easier.

AARP Caregiving Tools: www.aarp.org/caregivingtools

AARP's suite of web-based tools will help you find services, keep track of health recordsand more.

AARP Long-TermCare Cost Calculator: www.aarp.org/longtermcarecosts

Find and compare the costs of home care, assisted living and other services throughoutthe United States.

AARP Online Caregiving Community: www.aarp.org/caregivingcommunity

Join this community & connect with other caregiverslike you.

Administration on Community Living (ACL): www.acl.gov

The federal agency responsible for advancing the concerns and interests of older people. The website has a variety of tools and information for older adults and family caregivers.

Alzheimer's Association: www.alz.org or 800-272-3900

Resources, tools, anda 24-hour helpline for people with Alzheimer's disease and their families.

American Society on Aging

The American Society on Aging is a nonprofit organization committed to enhancing the knowledge and skills of those working with older adults and their families. Site offers useful resources on a variety of aging-related topics.

Website: http://www.asaging.org

American CancerSociety: www.cancer.org or 800-227-2345.

From basic information about cancer and its causes to in-depthinformation on specificcancer types— including risk factors, early detection, diagnosisand treatment options.

American DiabetesAssociation: www.diabetes.org or 800-342-2383

Resources and research to prevent, cure and manage diabetes.

American Heart Association: www.heart.org or 800-242-8721

Resources will help you better care for someone who has heart disease or who has had a heart attack,heart surgery or a stroke.

Care Advocates

Care Advocates provide guidance, support, and advocacy to families seeking care options such as residential care homes, assisted living facilities, and memory care facilities. They also offer comprehensive resources to address all of a family's care needs.

Website: https://advocatern.com

Care.com: www.care.com

Improving the lives of families and caregivers by helping them connect in a reliable and easy way.

Caregiver Action Network: www.caregiveraction.org or 202-454-3970

Information, educational materials and support for family caregivers.

Eldercare Care Resources: https://eldercare.acl.gov/Public/Search_Results.aspx

List of resources in your community that provide information and assistance for older adults and caregivers.

Eldercare Care Manager: https://advocatern.com/care-planning/

Elizabeth Dole Foundation: www.aarp.org/caregivingcommunity

Created to help American military caregivers by strengthening the services afforded to them through innovation, evidence-based research, and collaboration.

Family CaregiverAlliance: www.elizabethdolefoundation.org

Tools and resources for family caregivers, including the Family Care Navigator, a state-by-state list of services and assistance.

Food Assistance- local: ://covid19.sanantonio.gov/Resources/Food-Assistance

Tools and resources for family caregivers, including the Family Care Navigator, a state-by-state list of services and assistance.

LeadingAge: www.leadingage.org

Consumer information on long-term care facilities and services, and how to access them.

Loss of Life Advocates

LOLA's compassionate team offers the resources and assistance needed to navigate both the emotional and practical challenges you face. They help you prepare for the unexpected with thoughtful planning and personalized support.
Website: https://www.lossoflifeadvocates.com/

Medicade

Each state has rules about who is eligible for Medicaid and what it covers. Some people qualify for Medicaid, Medicare or both. Find out if you're eligible for Medicaid in Texas.

Website: https://yourtexasbenefits.com/Learn/Home

Medicare: **www.medicare.gov or 800-633-4227**

Provides information about the Medicare program and how to find Medicare plans and providers. Caregivers will also find a tool on the website to compare home health care agencies and nursing homes. The official U.S. government site for Medicare.

National Council on the Aging

The National Council on the Aging is an association of organizations and professionals dedicated to promoting the dignity, self-determination, well being, and contributions of older persons. The For Older Adults section of the site contains health related resources and tips. Website: **http://www.ncoa.org**

National Academy of Elder Law Attorneys: **www.naela.org**

A professional association of attorneys who specialize in legal services for older adults and people with special needs. Find information on legal issues affecting older adults and a database of elder law attorneys by state.

National Alliance for Caregiving: **www.caregiving.org**

This organization is dedicated to improving the quality of life for caregivers and those they care for through research, innovation and advocacy.

National Alliancefor Hispanic Health:

www.healthyamericas.org or 866-783-2645

The Hispanic Family Health Helpline and its Su Familia provide free and confidential health information for Hispanic families.

National Association for Home Care & Hospice: **www.nahc.org**

Consumer information on how to select a home care provider or hospice.

National Association of Home Builders:

A web-based directory of certified aging-in-place specialists who can identify and/or provide home modifications that make a home accessible, safer and more comfortable.
www.nahb.org/caps or 800-368-5242

National Hospice and PalliativeCare Organization

Provides free consumer information on hospice care and puts the public in direct contact with hospice programs.
www.nhpco.org or 800-646-6460

National Multiple Sclerosis Society: **www.nationalmssociety.org**

Offers resourcesand support to navigate the best life through the challenges of MS.

National ParkinsonFoundation: **www.parkinson.org or 800-473-4636**

Events, research progress and resources for those affected by Parkinson's disease.

National Respite Network: **www.archrespite.org**

A service that helps people locate respite services.

OASIS

San Antonio Oasis promotes healthy aging through lifelong learning, active lifestyles and volunteer engagement.

Website: https://san-antonio.oasisnet.org

Senior Centers

The senior Serives Division helps San Antonio older adult community lead an aciatve, indepenend and engaged lives thorught comprehensive nutrition helath wellness education and more.

Webiste:

https://www.sa.gov/Directory/Departments/DHS/Senior-Services/Senior-Centers

Social SecurityAdministration: www.ssa.gov or 800-772-1213

Help and information on eligibility and benefits,

State Health Insurance Assistance Program (SHIP):

Website: www.shiptacenter.org or 877-839-2675
A service that helps people locate respite services.

Texas Health and Human Services Aging Services

Resources, Benefits, Support
https://www.hhs.texas.gov/services/aging

The Conversation Project: www.theconversationproject.org

Created to help people talk about their wishes for end-of-life care.

Veterans Affairs: www.caregiver.va.gov or 855-260-3274

Support and services are available for caregivers of veterans. Provides local caregiver support for veterans.

2-1-1: www.211.org

A free and confidential service that helps people across North America find the local resources they need.

WORKSHEET

GOALS & NEEDS CHECKLIST

This list can be used to begin a discussion about the most important things to you and your loved ones, as well as their strengths..

Goals	Strengths
☐ To remain healthy and active	☐ Able to do most things on my own
☐ To stay/move near family	☐ Adequate savings and/or income
☐ To remain in my own home with care if needed	☐ Low-maintenance single-story home
☐ To move into independent living or assisted living	☐ Family and friends nearby
☐ To maintain hobbies	☐ Relationships with family
☐ To be around people	☐ Able to advocate for my self
☐ To move to a more accessible home (one story or apartment with elevator)	☐ Strong support system around me
☐ To be financially secure and/or to budget for future needs	☐ Able to drive
☐ To travel/visit home country	☐ Able to access resources
☐ Other	☐ Able to access emergency numbers
☐ Other	☐ Other
☐ Other	☐ Other

Your needs. Your loved ones needs

Determine if there is an urgent need. Prioritize the tasks and create a schedule.

GENERAL NEEDS ASSESSMENT

Area of Need	Types of PossibleTasks	Point Person
Home Maintenance and Living Situation	☐ Pay rent/mortgage	
	☐ Home repairs/modifications	
	☐ Safety concerns	
	☐ Grocery shopping & meal preparation	
	☐ Lawn care	
	☐ Pet care	
	☐ Housekeeping	
	☐ Research alternative living situations	
	☐ Research resources that can come into the home	
	☐ Home- Home care, visiting practitioners, therapies, podiatry	
Financial Affairs	☐ Paying bills	
	☐ Keeping track of financial records	
	☐ Managing assets	
	☐ Applying for and supervising public benefits	
Transportation Needs	☐ Driving decisions	
	☐ Coordinating rides	
	☐ Locating transportation services	
Personal Care	☐ Coordinating personal care activities	
	☐ Help with daily grooming and dressing	
	☐ Personal care outside the home	
	☐ Clothes shopping	

Area of Need	Types of PossibleTasks	Point Person
Health Care	☐ Monitor and recordphysical and emotional symptoms	
	☐ Arrange medical appointments, transportation, and someone to accompany as needed	
	☐ Submit medical insurance and bills	
	☐ Explain medical decisions	
	☐ Medication management (fill prescriptions, fill pill boxes, give reminders and dispense medications)	
	☐ Arrange for medical care in the home- therapies, visiting practitioners, podiatry, labs, etc.	
	☐ Obtain medical bracelet and/or medical alert system if needed	
	☐ Medical alert device	
Communications	☐ Paying bills	
	☐ Keeping track of financial records	
	☐ Daily check-in	
	☐ Obtain cell phone and/or Internet to	
	☐ enhance communication	
Socialization	☐ Coordinate social events	
	☐ Arranging for visitors	
	☐ Arranging outings	
Adaptive Devices	☐ Evaluating need for adaptive devices	
	☐ Training on how to use devices	
	☐ Other	
	☐ Other	

PERSONAL INFORMATION CHECKLIST

Name. ______________________________

X	Personal Information	Where Is It Kept? (attach copy of documents)	Contact Name
☐	Drivers License/ Donor Card		
☐	Birth Certificate		
☐	Marriage Certificate		
☐	Death Certificate (for deceased spouse)		
☐	Divorce Papers		
☐	Military Records • branch of service VA ID#: • discharge papers:		
☐	Social Security Card		
☐	Passport/Citizenship Papers		
☐	Address Books (names and addresses of friends and colleagues)		
☐	Lists of church & community memberships and contact information		
☐	Information on funeral arrangements		
☐	Pet care		
☐	Lawyer contact information		
☐	CPA / bookkeeper contact information		
☐	Other		

HOME MAINTENANCE CHECKLIST

X	Home Item	Where Is It Kept? (attach copy of documents)	Contact Name
☐	Mortgage Company Name: Amount due:		
☐	Rental Management Company: Amount due:		
☐	Rental/Real Estate Agent:		
☐	Gas/Electric/Water Company:		
☐	Cable/Internet/Telephone:		
☐	Home Security Company:		
☐	Home maintenance services.		
☐	Neighbor's Contact Information		
☐	Homeowners Insurance Agent: Insurance Policy #: Homeowners Premium:		
☐	Garbage Service/Garbage Pickup Day is: **M T W Th F (circle)** Recycle Service Pickup Day is: **M T W Th F (circle)**		
☐	Home Services: • Handy person • Lawn care • Appliances		
☐	Passwords • Computer(s) password clue(s) • Phone messages password clue		

MEDICAL CHECKLIST

PHARMACY Name	
PHONE #	
LOCATION	

PHARMACY Name	
PHONE #	
LOCATION	

DOCTOR Name/ Specialty	
PHONE #	
ADDRESS	

DOCTOR Name/ Specialty	
PHONE #	
ADDRESS	

DOCTOR Name/ Specialty	
PHONE #	
ADDRESS	

DOCTOR Name	
PHONE #	
ADDRESS	

DOCTOR Name	
PHONE #	
ADDRESS	

DENTIST Name	
PHONE #	
ADDRESS	

HOME CARE AGENCY	
PHONE #	
ADDRESS	

OTHER AGENCY	
PHONE #	
ADDRESS	

MEDICAL CHECKLIST (continued)

X	Item	Where Is It Kept?	Contact Name
☐	Medicare Originalor MedicareAdvantage (company name): ID Number:		
☐	Medicare Prescription Drug Coverage (company name): ID Number: (does not apply to an Advantage plan with drug coverage)		
☐	Other Health Insurance Policy (Medigap): Company: Premium: Payment schedule		
☐	Veterans Health System: ID Number:		
☐	Do Not Resuscitate (DNR) Order:		
☐	Physician Orders for Life-Sustaining Treatment (POLST) form— if availablein your state		
☐	Living Will/Advance Directives/ Attorney information.		
☐	Durable Power of Attorney for Health Care		
☐	Other end of life forms		
☐	Other important documents related to medical care		

LIST OF MEDICATIONS

Prescription Name	Strength	Dosage	Warnings/ Instructions

TRANSPORTION CHECKLIST

X	Item	Notes	Where Is It Kept?
☐	Auto(s):	Make(s):	
☐	Auto Loan Information:	Model(s):	
☐	Title for Car(s):		
☐	Auto Insurance Company:		
☐	Recreational Vehicles: Title: Insurance:		
☐	Transportation Services (such as ACCESS van or local cab service):		
☐	Transportation assistance from friends and famly- list names and contact numbers		

FINANCIAL ITEM CHECKLIST

BENEFITS CHECKLIST

X	Personal Information	Where Is It Kept?	Contact Name
☐	Banking information (checking/savings accounts) Pin number clues — online banking and accounts with passwords and clues		
☐	Trusts		
☐	Will		
☐	Durable Power of Attorney for Finances		
☐	Any Rental Agreements or Business Contracts		
☐	Complete List of Assets & Debts		
☐	Household bills		
☐	Federal & State Tax Returns (past 3-5 years): Tax Preparer		
☐	Records of Any Personal Loans Made to Others:		
☐	Financial Planner or Broker:		
☐	Life Insurance Policy or Policies:		
☐	Disability Insurance (long- and short-term):		
☐	Long-Term Care Insurance:		
☐	Safe Deposit Box(es):		

BENEFITS CHECKLIST

If you or a loved one is eligible, you may be able to get help paying for your food, heating bills or property taxes.

Find out what programs are available in your state go to https://advocatern.com/resources/

X	Item	
☐	Food Assistance (i.e., SNAP/FNS)	YES ☐ - NO ☐
☐	Low Income Home Energy Assistance (LIHEAP)	YES ☐ - NO ☐
☐	Supplemental Security Income (SSI)	YES ☐ - NO ☐
☐	Property Tax Assistance	YES ☐ - NO ☐
☐	Extra Help Paying for Medicare Part D (prescription drug coverage)	YES ☐ - NO ☐
☐	Medicare Parts A, B, and D Premium Support	YES ☐ - NO ☐
☐	Medicaid (help with long-term care and medical care) Number & Identification Card	YES ☐ - NO ☐

SAMPLE CAREGIVING PLAN

Caregiving plans can be as simple or detailed as your team and you desire. This simple plan can be used to decide together on the goals, actions, responsible person and timing. Include a goal of self-care for you and your team.

Name : ______________________ Date Started: ______________

Team Members: ______________________________________

Contact Info: ______________________________________

Need	Steps	Person Responsible	Timeframe
1. Better understand and manage dads care needs	**We will meet with dad and his doctors** • Create list of medications to be taken • Organize medications in pill box • Organize appointment in calendars • dSet appointments for dad • Who will take dad to doctor • Take notes at each appointment in journal and get written instructions from doctor • Confirm follow-up/appointments		
2. Coordinate home resources for dad	• Determine care and resources needed, • Outline the resources; Visiting practitioners, podiatry, therapies, etc. • Interview these resources and care that will come into the home • Arrange schedule		
3. Coordinate dads outside visits to doctors and personal errands:	• Find out what appointments dad has. • Create Schedule. • assign these appointments and trasnporstation.		

SAMPLE DETAILED FOR TASKS

Daily task schedule Caregiving Week of: ____________________

Day	Tasks	When	Person(s) Responsible	Timeframe
Monday	• Check if medications have been taken • Go to doctor's appt	End of day 1:00 p.m.	Daughter Mary Daughter Ann	Call and review pill box Drive to appt, get prescriptions, set in pill box
Tuesday	• Go grocery shopping • Check on medications • Check if any supplies are needed	After work	Son Al	Call Mom for grocery list at lunch, shop after work and drop over. Check pill box when dropping off groceries. Look in fridge for spoiled food
Wednesday	• Confirm all appointments for the month	End of day	Daughter Mary	Call and review pill box
Thursday	• Check on home-delivered meals on the holiday • Check on medications	Today End of day	Daughter Mary Daughter Mary	Call agency to see if meals will be delivered next Monday Call and review pill box
Friday	• Check on medical bill payment • Delegate who will bring in lunch and dinner for the weekend.	Today	Daughter Mary	Make call to insurance provider about payment Call Peggy to fill in for Monday lunch
Saturday	• Clean and do laundry • Drive to beauty parlor • Check on medications	Afternoon	Daughter Ann	Make call to insurance provider about payment Call Peggy to fill in for Monday lunch
Sunday	• Do Medication box • Take to faithservices • Arrange for visitor oroutings and calancer for the week	Evening 9:00 a.m. 1:00 p.m	Mary Al Niece Beth	Review medications and place in pill box for the week Drive Mom to service

CARE ADVOCATES™
CARE OPTIONS • SENIOR PLACEMENT

RESOURCES

ADVOCACY

GUIDANCE

SUPPORT

210-669-2222

www.advocatern.com

laura@advocatern.com

Laura Daniels, RN

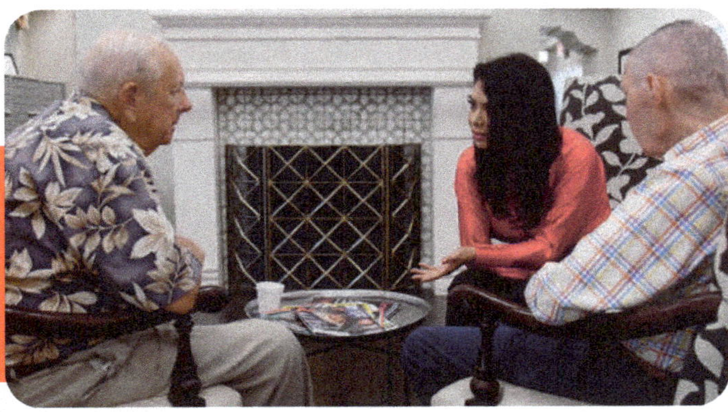

www.ingramcontent.com/pod-product-compliance
Lightning Source LLC
LaVergne TN
LVHW060045210926
848481LV00013B/3955
* 9 7 9 8 3 4 9 3 7 8 5 2 2 *